The Complete Mediterranean Dash Diet Recipe Book

Tasty and Affordable Mediterranean Dash Diet Recipes to Start Your Day with the Right Foot

Kathyrn Solano

© Copyright 2021 - All rights reserved.

The content contained within this book may not be reproduced, duplicated or transmitted without direct written permission from the author or the publisher.

Under no circumstances will any blame or legal responsibility be held against the publisher, or author, for any damages, reparation, or monetary loss due to the information contained within this book. Either directly or indirectly.

Legal Notice:

This book is copyright protected. This book is only for personal use. You cannot amend, distribute, sell, use, quote or paraphrase any part, or the content within this book, without the consent of the author or publisher.

Disclaimer Notice:

Please note the information contained within this document is for educational and entertainment purposes only. All effort has been executed to present accurate, up to date, and reliable, complete information. No warranties of any kind are declared or implied. Readers acknowledge that the author is not engaging in the rendering of legal, financial, medical or professional advice. The content within this book has been derived from various sources. Please consult a licensed professional before attempting any techniques outlined in this book.

By reading this document, the reader agrees that under no circumstances is the author responsible for any losses, direct or indirect, which are incurred as a result of the use of information contained within this document, including, but not limited to, — errors, omissions, or inaccuracies.

Table of contents

GREAT MEDITERRANEAN DIET RECIPES 6
    Muesli muffins 6
    Panforte 8
    Pear and crumble 10
    Simple warm fruit dessert 12
    Banana Ice-cream 14
    Spicy bean cake 15
    Berry breakfast smoothie 17
    Bircher muesli with apple & banana 18
    Buckwheat pancakes 19
    Mushroom & Spinach Omelets 20
    Raspberry strawberry smoothie 22
    Porridge (Oatmeal) 23
    Fattoush Salad 25
    Poached Eggs Caprese 27
    Eggs and Greens Breakfast Dish 29
    Breakfast Pita Pizza 30
    Caprese on Toast 32
    Quinoa Breakfast Cereal 33
    Zucchini with Egg 34
    Scrumptious Breakfast Salad 35
    Blueberry Lemon Breakfast Quinoa 37
    Cheesy Artichoke and Spinach Frittata 38
    Strawberries in Balsamic Yogurt Sauce 40
    Spinach Feta Breakfast Wraps 41
    Easy, Fluffy Lemon Ricotta Pancakes 42
    Smashed Egg Toasts with Herby Lemon Yogurt 43
    Avocado and Egg Breakfast Pizza 45
    Avocado milkshake 47
    Pumpkin oatmeal with spices 48
    Creamy oatmeal with figs 49
    Breakfast spanakopita 50
    Stuffed figs 51
    Vegetable breakfast bowl 52
    Breakfast green smoothie 53
    Simple and quick steak 54
    Vegetable stew 55
    Hot curry powder 57

- Low sodium mayonnaise 58
- Green breakfast soup 59
- Creamy broccoli soup 60
- Roasted root vegetables 61
- Spinach falafel wrap 62
- Vegetable biryani 64
- Greek couscous salad 66
- German braised cabbage 67
- Vibrant carrot soup 68
- Open-faced bagel breakfast sandwich 69
- Rigatoni with emerald sauce 70
- Korean mushroom bibimbap 71
- Bulgur wheat salad with pomegranate molasses chicken 73
- Broccoli and Capsicum Pasta Salad 75
- Sesame Salad Dressing 77
- Mediterranean Grain Salad 78
- Macadamia Nut Dressing 79
- Vinaigrette Dressing 80
- Steamed Broccoli Salad 81
- Pomegranate Feta Salad 82
- Grated beetroot & carrot salad 84
- Roasted vegetable lentil salad 86
- Herbed Quinoa and Pomegranate Salad 88
- Salad Niçoise 90
- Roasted sweet potato and black bean salad 92
- Cannellini Bean Soup 94
- Garlic, sweet potato, and chickpea soup 96
- Kumara, coconut, and lemongrass soup 97
- Moroccan Chickpea Soup 99
- Ribollita 100
- Broccoli soup 102
- Mushroom soup 104
- Guacamole 106
- Mushroom & Cardamom, Squash Soup 107

GREAT MEDITERRANEAN DIET RECIPES

Muesli muffins

Preparation time: 10 minutes
Cooking time: 25 minutes
Servings: 7

Ingredients:
100 g flour
2 tsp baking powder
50 g plain flour
1/2 tsp cinnamon
One pinch salt
Two eggs
100 g muesli
35 g milk
100 g butter
100 g panela sugar
100 ml of milk
1 tsp vanilla extract

Directions:

Preheat the oven to 400 degrees. Take the butter and melt it in a pan.

Now mix the dry ingredients. A large bowl adds the two flours, baking powder, ground cinnamon, muesli, orange zest, sugar, salt, and chocolate chips.

Mix the wet ingredients with dry. In another bowl, add the milk, eggs, and vanilla. Beat the eggs with the milk by using a fork. Now add the cooled butter and mix it again.

Load the muffin cases with more muesli. Cover the cases with the batter mixture using a cake spoon. You want them to be half to two-thirds complete. You will plan to measure each muffin to ensure the same amount. Any of them would weigh around 90g. Taking a couple more of your chosen muesli. Delete the dried fruit from the (placing it back in your cereal container). Spread the oats, seeds, and nuts over the top of the raw muffins.

Bake it for 25 min. You have to change the direction of the tray every 18 min. Allow the muffins to rest on a cooling rack.

Nutrition Info: Calories: 380 kcal Fat:20 g Protein:7 g Carbs: 45 g Fiber: 2 g

Panforte

Preparation time: 20 minutes
Cooking time: 40 minutes
Servings: 20 slices

Ingredients:

3/4 cup roasted almonds

1.5 cup candied fruit

3/4 tsp nutmeg

3/4 whole hazelnuts roasted

3 tbsp honey

1 cup granulated sugar

1 tbsp water

1 cup flour

3/4 tsp coriander powder

1 tsp cinnamon

3/4 tsp ground cloves

1 tbsp icing sugar

Directions:

Preheat oven to 300 degrees. Spray the cake pan with oil.
In a mixing bowl, mix the nuts and candied fruit. In a medium skillet, whisk the flour and flavors.
In a small pan, mix honey, water, and sugar, heat on medium flame with continuous stirring till the mixture starts to boil, lower the slow heat boiling for 2-3 min.

Add the honey mixture to the nut mixture and mix them. Add the flour mixture and quickly stir.

Put the batter into the prepared cake pan and with wet hands. Dust the top with a tbsp of icing sugar before baking. Bake it for 35 to 40 min.

Let the cake cool for 10 to 15 min. Place it on a cake stand and make it cool and dust with icing sugar. Took a piece with a sharp knife and enjoyed it!

Nutrition Info: Calories: 196 kcal Fat:5 g Protein:3 g Carbs: 36 g Fiber: 2 g

Pear and crumble

Preparation time:10 minutes
Cooking time: 45 minutes
Servings: 6

Ingredients:

Crumble topping

200 g flour

100 g ground almonds

100 g butter

75 g caster sugar

Fruit filling

500 g plums

1 tsp corn flour

Two pears

3 tbsp caster sugar

Directions:

Preheat the oven to 18 degrees.

Put 200-gram flour, 100-gram butter,100-gram ground almonds, and 75-gram caster sugar into a food processor and blitz till the batter look a lot like crumbs. On the other hand, spread the butter into the flour until the mixture looks like uneven breadcrumbs. Add the almonds and sugar and set it down.

To make the filling

Rinse 500g plums, cut into quarters dumping the stones, and place in a narrow baking tray. Peel, core, and thickly slice two pears add to the dish. Season with 1 tsp corn flour and 3 tbsp caster sugar and mix it.

To complete

Place the fruit level in the dish and dress over the crushed topping. Put the dish on a baking sheet and bake until golden.

Nutrition Info: Calories: 480 kcal Fat:22 g Protein:8 g Carbs: 66 g Fiber: 6 g

Simple warm fruit dessert

Preparation time: 10 minutes
Cooking time: 60 minutes
Servings: 6

Ingredients:

Three sliced Apples
½ tsp Lemon juiced
Three cored & sliced pears
1 tsp Ground Cinnamon
½ tbsp Orange Zest
2 Cup Grapes
1/4 tsp Ground Nutmeg
2 cup cranberries
1 Orange Juiced
1/3 cup Maple Syrup
2 tbsp Coconut Oil

Directions:

Preheat the oven to 300 degrees and spray it with coconut oil. Mix apples and pears in a bowl. Add lemon zest, cinnamon, nutmeg, and toss the fruits with a spoon to coat with the juice. Shift the fruits in the baking dish & add in grapes and cranberries.
In a mixing bowl, whisk fresh orange zest, Apple syrup, and coconut oil. Put the dressing over the fruits.

Bake it in the oven for one hour. Once the fruits are done, remove them from the oven and let them cool at room temperature.
Season with some cinnamon and serve.

Nutrition Info: Calories: 258 kcal Fat: 5 g Protein:1 g Carbs:57 g Fiber:8 g

Banana Ice-cream

Preparation time: 3 minutes

Cooking time: 0 minute

Servings: 1

Ingredients:

2 tbsp peanut butter

Two frozen bananas

5 tbsp almond milk

Directions:

In a blender, mix the bananas and the milk.

Once they are partly chopped up, add in the nut butter.

Nutrition Info: Calories: 125 kcal Fat: 0.4 g Protein:1.3 g Carbs:26.9 g Fiber: 3.1 g

Spicy bean cake

Preparation time: 20 minutes
Cooking time: 15 minutes
Servings: 8

Ingredients:
Lime Sour Cream
1/2cup cream reduced-fat sour
One jalapeno pepper
2 tbsp lime juice
Salt to taste
Bean Cake
2 tbsp olive oil
Six garlic cloves
Four green onions
Two jalapeno peppers
Two cans of black beans
1 tbsp cumin
salt & black pepper to taste
One egg
2 cup grated potato
½ cup bread crumb

Directions:
Mix the lime cream, jalapeno, and salt in a small bowl

Cook green onions in 1 tbsp olive oil until softened, about 1 minute. Add garlic, two diced jalapenos, and cumin; heat until aromatic, for 30 sec.

Shift it to skillet. Mix in black beans, and mash with a fork. Dress with salt and pepper. Mix in sweet potatoes, egg, and bread crumbs. Split into eight balls and compressed into patties. In the oven, set the cooking rack about 4 inches from the heat source. Grease baking sheet with 1 tbsp oil.

Put bean patties on a baking sheet, and broil 8 to 10 min. Serve with sour lime cream.

Nutrition Info: Calories: 218kcal Fat: 6.7 g Protein: 9.4 g Carbs: 31.3 g Fiber: 0 g

Berry breakfast smoothie

Preparation time: 5 minutes

Cooking time: 5 minutes

Servings: 2

Ingredients:

2 cup milk

1/2 cup oats

2 cup berries

2 tsp chia seeds

Directions:

Add milk with fruit and oats in a blender.

Blend it smoothly, mix in chia seeds and serve instantly.

Nutrition Info: Calories:117 kcal Fat: 1 g Protein: 8 g Carbs:18 g Fiber: 4 g

Bircher muesli with apple & banana

Preparation time: 5 minutes
Cooking time: chilling time -minutes
Servings: 2

Ingredients:

25 g organic sultanas
One grated apple
25 g seeds (sunflower, pumpkin, sesame, and linseed)
50 goats
25 g nuts chopped
100 g yogurt
1/4 tsp cinnamon
One sliced medium banana

Directions:

Add the grated apple in a bowl and add the oats, seeds, half the nuts, and cinnamon. Stir it well. Whisk yogurt & water, and chill it overnight.

Nutrition Info: Calories: 405 kcal Fat: 18 g Protein: g Carbs: g Fiber: g

Buckwheat pancakes

Preparation time: 10 minutes
Cooking time: 11 minutes
Servings: 4

Ingredients:
1/4 tsp vanilla extract 1 cup buckwheat flour
1 tsp baking powder 1.5 tsp sugar
1/4 tsp salt
1.25 cup buttermilk
1/4 tsp baking powder
One egg
1 tbsp butter

Directions:
Whisk wet ingredients in one bowl and dry in another.
Then mix the content of both the bowl.
Cook batter in melted butter for five minutes.

Nutrition Info: Calories: 196.4 kcal Fat: 5.8g Protein: 9.1 g Carbs: 25.7 g Fiber: 6 g

Mushroom & Spinach Omelets

Preparation time: 15 minutes

Cooking time: 15 minutes

Servings: 2

Ingredients:

One egg

1 cup spinach

1 tbsp shredded Parmesan cheese

Three egg whites

1 tbsp grated Cheddar cheese

1/8 tsp red pepper flakes

1/4 tsp salt

1/8 tsp garlic powder

1/8 tsp black pepper

1/8 tsp nutmeg

1/2 tsp olive oil

1/4 cup green onion

1/2 cup sliced mushrooms

2 tbsp red bell pepper

1/2 cup tomato

Directions:

Beat egg and egg whites in a bowl. Mix in cheese, salt, flakes, garlic, nutmeg, and pepper.

Heat oil in skillet; cook and stir mushrooms, onion, and pepper for 5 min. Put spinach in a skillet and cook. Add the egg and tomato mixture in it and keep cooking till it sets on top. Once done, cut into pieces, and serve instantly.

Nutrition Info: Calories: 114.4 kcal Fat:5.1 g Protein: 12.5 g Carbs: 5.7 g Fiber: 1.8 g

Raspberry strawberry smoothie

Preparation time: 10 minutes

Cooking time: 10 minutes

Servings: 1

Ingredients:

1 tbsp honey

1 cup hulled fresh strawberries

½ cup milk

½ cup raspberries

½ cup vanilla yogurt

1 tsp vanilla extract

Directions: Put all the ingredients in a blender and blend until a smooth consistency is attained.

Nutrition Info: Calories: 317.7 kcal Fat: 4.7 g Protein: 11.7 g Carbs: 58.6 g Fiber: 7.1 g

Porridge (Oatmeal)

Preparation time: 2 minutes
Cooking time: 2 minutes
Servings: 1

Ingredients:
Base Recipe
½ cup oats
1/2cup water
1/2cup milk
1 Pinch salt
Maple Brown Sugar
1 tsp sugar
2 tbsp chopped pecans
1 tsp maple syrup
1/8 tsp cinnamon
Banana Nut
½ banana sliced
1 tbsp flaxseed
2 tbsp walnuts
1/8 tsp cinnamon
Strawberry & Cream
1/2cup strawberries
2 tsp honey
1 tbsp half and half
1/8 tsp vanilla extract

Chocolate Peanut Butter

2 tsp cocoa powder

2 tsp chocolate chips

1 tbsp peanut butter

1 tsp roasted peanuts

Directions:

Microwave Instructions

Place all the ingredients heat in the microwave on high for 2 minutes. Then add 15-sec increments until the oatmeal is puffed and softened. Stovetop Instructions.

Bring the water and milk to a boil in a pan. Lower the heat & pour in the oats. Cook it while stirring, till the oats are soft and have absorbed most of the liquid. Turn off the stove and let it for 2 to 3 min. Assembly. Stir in the toppings and let rest for a few minutes to cool. Serve warm.

Nutrition Info: Calories: 227 kcal Fat:6 g Protein: 9 g Carbs: 33 g Fiber: 4 g

Fattoush Salad

Preparation time: 20 minutes
Cooking time: 20 minutes
Servings: 6

Ingredients:
- Two loaves of pita bread
- ½ tsp sumac
- Olive Oil
- Salt and pepper
- One chopped English cucumber
- One chopped lettuce
- Five chopped Roma tomatoes
- Five radishes
- Five chopped green onions
- 2 cup parsley leaves

Lime-vinaigrette
- 1/4 tsp cinnamon
- 1 tsp lime juice
- Salt and pepper
- 1/3 cup Virgin Olive Oil
- 1 tsp sumac
- 1/4 tsp allspice

Directions:

Toast the bread in the oven. Heat olive oil and fry until browned. Add salt, pepper, and 1/2tsp of sumac. Turn off heat & place pita chips on paper towels to drain.

In a mixing bowl, mix the chopped lettuce, cucumber, tomatoes, green onions with the sliced radish and parsley.

For seasoning, whisk the lemon or lime juice, olive oil, and spices in a small bowl.

Sprinkle the salad & toss lightly. Finally, add the pita chips and more sumac if you like. Shifts to small serving bowls or plates. Enjoy!

Nutrition Info: Calories: 345 kcal Fat:20.4 g Protein: 9.1 g Carbs:39.8 g Fiber: 1 g

Poached Eggs Caprese

Preparation time:10 minutes

Cooking time: 10 minutes

Servings: 2

Ingredients:

- 4 tsp pesto
- 1 tbsp white vinegar
- Four eggs
- 2 tsp salt
- 2 English muffins
- salt to taste
- One tomato sliced
- Four slices of mozzarella cheese

Directions:

Fill 2 to 3 inches of a pan with water and boil over a high flame. Lower the heat, add the vinegar, 2 tsp of salt in it, and let it simmer.

Put a cheese slice and a slice of tomato on every English muffin half and put in a toaster oven for 5 min or till the cheese melts and the English muffin is well toasted.

Break an egg in a bowl and add in the water one by one. Let the eggs cook for 2.5 to 3 minutes or until the yolks have solidified and the egg whites are firm. Take the eggs out of the water and put them on a kitchen towel to absorb excess water.

For assembling, first put an egg on top of every muffin, add a tsp of pesto sauce on the egg, and scatter the salt.

Nutrition Info: Calories: 482.1 kcal Fat: g Protein: 33.3 g Carbs: 31.7 g Fiber:1.2 g

Eggs and Greens Breakfast Dish

Preparation time: 10 minutes
Cooking time: 10 minutes
Servings: 2

Ingredients:
- 1 tbsp olive oil
- salt to taste
- 2 cup chopped rainbow chard
- ½ cup arugula
- 1 cup spinach
- Two cloves garlic
- ½ cup grated Cheddar cheese
- Four eggs
- black pepper to taste

Directions:
Heat oil over moderate pressure. Sauté the chard, spinach, and arugula until soft, around three minutes. Add garlic, continue cooking until aromatic, approx. Two min.
In a cup, combine the eggs and the cheese; dump into the mixture of the chard. Heat and cook for 5 - 6 minutes. Season to taste with salt and pepper.

Nutrition Info: Calories:332.5 kcal Fat: 26.2 g Protein: 21 g Carbs:4.2 g Fiber: 1 g

Breakfast Pita Pizza

Preparation time: 25 minutes
Cooking time: 30 minutes
Servings: 2

Ingredients:
- Four slices of bacon
- 2 tbsp olive oil
- 1/4 onion
- Four eggs
- Two pita bread rounds
- 2 tbsp pesto
- ½ tomato
- One avocado
- ½ cup slashed spinach
- 1/4 cup mushrooms
- ½ cup grated Cheddar cheese

Directions:
Heat the oven to 350 ° F (175° C).
In a medium saucepan, put the bacon and cook over medium-high heat, rotating periodically, when browned uniformly, around ten minutes. Cook the onion in the same skillet till smooth. Put it aside. In the skillet, melt the olive oil. Add the eggs and cook, stirring regularly, for 3 to 5 minutes. Add the pita bread to the cake pan. Cover with bacon, fried eggs, onions,

mushrooms, and spinach; sprinkle the pesto over through the pita. Dress over the toppings of Cheddar cheese.

Bake it in the preheated oven for10 min. Serve with avocado pieces.

Nutrition Info: Calories: 873.2 kcal Fat: 62 g Protein: 36.8 g Carbs:43.5 g Fiber: 9.5 g

Caprese on Toast

Preparation time: 15 minutes
Cooking time: 5 minutes
Servings: 14

Ingredients:
- 14 slices bread
- 1 lb mozzarella cheese
- Two cloves garlic
- 1/3 cup basil leaves
- 3 tbsp olive oil
- Three tomatoes
- salt to taste
- black pepper to taste

Directions: Baked the bread slices and spread the garlic on one side of each piece. Put a slice of mozzarella cheese, 1 to 2 basil leaves, and a slice of tomato on each piece of toast. Sprinkle with olive oil, spray salt, and black pepper.

Nutrition Info: Calories: 203.5 kcal Fat: 10 g Protein: 10.5 g Carbs: 16.5 g Fiber: 1.1 g

Quinoa Breakfast Cereal

Preparation time: 5 minutes
Cooking time: 16 minutes
Servings: 4

Ingredients:
- 2 cups of water
- ½ cup apricots
- 1 cup quinoa
- ½ cup almonds
- 1 tsp cinnamon
- 1/3 cup seeds
- ½ tsp nutmeg

Directions: Combine water and quinoa in a medium saucepan and continue cooking. Lower the heat and boil when much of the water has been drained for 8–12 minutes. Whisk in apricots, almonds, linseeds, cinnamon, and nutmeg; simmer till the quinoa is soft.

Nutrition Info: Calories: 349.9 kcal Fat:15.1 g Protein: 11.8 g Carbs: 44.5 g Fiber: 9.3 g

Zucchini with Egg

Preparation time: 5 minutes
Cooking time: 15 minutes
Servings: 2

Ingredients:
- Two eggs
- 1.5 tbsp olive oil
- salt to taste
- Two zucchinis
- Black pepper to taste
- 1 tsp water

Directions: Heat the oil in a saucepan over medium heat; sauté the zucchini until soft, around 10 minutes. Season with salt and black pepper.
Add the eggs with a fork in a bowl; add more water and mix until uniformly mixed. Spill the eggs over the zucchini; continue cooking until the eggs are boiled and rubbery for almost 5 minutes. Dress it with salt and black pepper.

Nutrition Info: Calories: 21.7 kcal Fat: 15.7 g Protein: 10.2 g Carbs: 11.2 g Fiber: 3.6 g

Scrumptious Breakfast Salad

Preparation time: 35 minutes
Cooking time: 5 minutes
Servings: 4

Ingredients:
- Five eggs
- Two avocados
- One head romaine lettuce
- Two tomatoes
- Four clementine
- 1-pint strawberries
- One onion
- One cucumber
- One apple
- One peeled mango
- One nectarine
- 1/4 cup vinaigrette

Directions:
Boil eggs in a pan. Turn off the flame. Let the eggs rest in hot water for 15 min.
Cover spinach, avocados, tomatoes, strawberries, clementine, cabbage, peach, apple, nectarine, and cucumber in a large mixing bowl or on an individual platter. Sprinkle the vinaigrette at the tip.

Take eggs from hot water; cool in ice water. Peel it and chop it. Spread the eggs over the salad.

Nutrition Info: Calories: 447.5 kcal Fat: 24.2 g Protein:13.4 g Carbs: 53.7 g Fiber: 15.6 g

Blueberry Lemon Breakfast Quinoa

Preparation time: 5 minutes

Cooking time: 25 minutes

Servings: 2

Ingredients:

- 3 tbsp maple syrup
- 1 cup quinoa
- One pinch salt
- ½ lemon
- 2 cup milk
- 1 cup blueberries
- 2 tsp flax seed

Directions: Wash quinoa in a fine sieve of ice water to extract bitterness when the water is pure and no stickier. Pour the milk into a pan over medium heat for 2 - 3 mins. Mix the quinoa and salt in the milk; boil over moderate heat once all of the liquid was being consumed, around twenty minutes. In the quinoa mixer, slowly fold the blueberries & add the apple and the lime juice. Serve quinoa mixture in 2 bowls; sprinkle 1 tsp linseed to eat.

Nutrition Info: Calories: 537.8 kcal Fat: 7.3 g Protein: 21.5 g Carbs: 98.7 g Fiber: 8.9 g

Cheesy Artichoke and Spinach Frittata

Preparation time: 5 minutes
Cooking time: 40 minutes
Servings: 8 slices

Ingredients:
- 3 tbsp pesto
- 1/2 cup milk
- 12 eggs
- 1/2 cup parmesan cheese, shredded
- 2 tsp olive oil
- 14.5 oz artichokes, chopped
- Two garlic cloves
- 1 cup cheese
- 6 cup baby spinach
- 1/2 tsp kosher salt

Directions:
Preheat the oven to 375 F.
Take a bowl and put milk, eggs, cheese, salt in it, and whisk together. Dry the artichokes using a paper towel. Take a skillet and heat olive oil in it over medium flame. Sauté the garlic in it for half a minute and put 4 cups of baby spinach in it. Cook them until they become soft, and then add the rest of the spinach in it with artichokes and sauté. Add the egg mixture to the skillet and reduce the flame to medium-low. Cook the eggs

for 1 minute without stirring. Once the eggs are cooked, stir it to mix well and top with leftover whole artichokes. Put the skillet in the preheated oven.

Bake for about 20 minutes or until its edges start to turn brown and puffed from the top.

Take out of the oven and put the pesto on it, and sprinkle with cheese. Bake for five more minutes or until the cheese melts, and a frittata is cooked thoroughly. Sprinkle the black pepper and fresh basil on top.

Nutrition Info: Calories: 234 kcal Fat: 16 g Protein: 16 g Carbs: 6 g Fiber: 2 g

Strawberries in Balsamic Yogurt Sauce

Preparation time: 15 minutes
Cooking time: 180 minutes
Servings: 3.2 oz

Ingredients:
- 1 tbsp honey
- 1 tbsp balsamic vinegar
- 1 cup sliced strawberries
- 1/2 cup yogurt

Directions: Mix all the ingredients in a bowl except strawberries. Put strawberries on top of each serving and refrigerate for 2-3 hours, then serve.

Nutrition Info: Calories: 51 kcal Fat: g Protein:3 g Carbs: 9 g Fiber:1 g

Spinach Feta Breakfast Wraps

Preparation time: 5 minutes
Cooking time: 5 minutes
Servings: 1

Ingredients:
Two eggs
4 Kalamata olives
1/2 cup spinach
1/4 cup feta cheese 1.5 tbsp butter
salt to taste
One tortilla
Black pepper to taste

Directions:
Gather the ingredients. Heat the pan to medium heat. Add 0.5of a tbsp of butter to the pan. Scramble the eggs in a small bowl. Add in the rest of the butter chunks and salt and pepper. Add the egg mixture to the pan. Let the eggs cook for a moment, add in the spinach and mix till the spinach and egg are cooked. Put eggs over the tortilla. Top the eggs with the feta cheese crumbles and chopped Kalamata olives.

Nutrition Info: Calories:399 kcal Fat: 22.9 g Protein: 19.6 g Carbs: 29.2 g Fiber: 2.3 g

Easy, Fluffy Lemon Ricotta Pancakes

Preparation time: 5 minutes
Cooking time: 20 minutes
Servings: 6

Ingredients:

1.25 cup ricotta cheese
Three eggs
One lemon
3/4 cup buttermilk
2 tbsp sugar
1 tbsp baking powder 1.25 cup flour
1/4 tsp sea salt
Olive oil

Directions: In a mixing bowl, whisk eggs and sugar. Add the buttermilk, salt, and ricotta cheese in it and whisk. In another bowl, mix flour and baking powder, then put it into the cheese mixture.
Heat a large non-stick skillet. Spoon batter into the pan. Repeat with the remaining batter.

Nutrition Info: Calories: 245 kcal Fat: 9 g Protein: 12 g Carbs: 28 g Fiber:1 g

Smashed Egg Toasts with Herby Lemon Yogurt

Preparation time: 4 minutes

Cooking time: 15 minutes

Servings: 4

Ingredients:

Eight eggs

One lemon

One clove garlic

Two fresh basil leaves

Four slices of bread

2 tbsp chives

2 tbsp dill

2 cup yogurt

3/4 tsp salt

2 tbsp olive oil

1/2 tsp black pepper

4 tbsp butter

Directions: Boil eight large eggs for exactly 6 minutes and 30 seconds. Let sit in the ice bath for 2 min, then peel the eggs and set aside.

In a medium bowl, mince one garlic clove, finely grate the zest one medium lemon, then juice the lemon. Finely chopped 2 tbsp fresh basil leaves, 2 tbsp fresh dill, and 2 tbsp fresh chives. Add

2 cup yogurt, 2 tbsp olive oil, 0.75 tsp kosher salt, and 0.5 tsp black pepper.

Cut four crusty bread. Melt 2 tbsp unsalted butter in a large skillet. Add 2 of the slices and cook until crispy, for 2 min per side. Shift to a large platter. Repeat with the remaining.

Place the yogurt and eggs on the bread. Drizzle salt and pepper and herbs with oil.

Nutrition Info: Calories: 437 kcal Fat: 35.5 g Protein: 23.5 g Carbs: 7.4 g Fiber: 0.6 g

Avocado and Egg Breakfast Pizza

Preparation time: 5 minutes
Cooking time: 40 minutes
Servings: 4

Ingredients:
1 Hass avocado
1 1/2 tsp lime juice
1 tbsp cilantro
1/8 tsp salt
Four eggs
1/2 lb pizza dough
1 tbsp vegetable oil

Directions:
Cut the avocado in halves using a spoon, but it's flesh in a bowl. Add the lime juice, cilantro, and salt. Mash well with a fork to form a smooth paste.
Divide the dough into four equal pieces. Roll each piece into a thin 6-inch circle.
Place one of the dough circles in the center of the skillet. Cook for 1- 2 min, until it is browned. Turn and cook another side until browned, pressing down with a spatula. Shift it to a plate and repeat.
Apply 0.5 of the avocado mixture onto each cooked slice of dough.

Fry eggs to desired doneness and place each one on top of a pizza. Serve immediately.

Nutrition Info: Calories: 337 kcal Fat: 17.6 g Protein: 12.3 g Carbs: 33.4 g Fiber: 4.9 g

Avocado milkshake

Preparation time: 10 minutes

Cooking time:10 minutes

Servings: 3

Ingredients:

1 cup milk

One banana

One avocado

3 tbsp honey

Directions:

Blend milk, avocado, banana, and honey in a blender until smooth

Nutrition Info: Calories: 246.7 kcal Fat: 11.6 g Protein: 4.5 g Carbs: 33.8 g Fiber: 5.6 g

Pumpkin oatmeal with spices

Preparation time: 3minutes

Cooking time:3 minutes

Servings: 1

Ingredients:

1/2 cup water

½ cup dried oats

2 tbsp pumpkin puree

½ cup unsweetened almond milk

1/2 tsp pure vanilla extract

1 tbsp maple syrup

1/4 tsp pumpkin pie spice

Directions: Mix all the ingredients in a bow. Microwave them for three minutes.

Nutrition Info: Calories: 243kcal Fat:4 g Protein: 6g Carbs: 44g Fiber:5 g

Creamy oatmeal with figs

Preparation time: minutes
Cooking time: minutes
Servings: 3

Ingredients:
1 tbsp light butter
1 tbsp honey
Five whole figs
1 cup rolled oats
1 cup low fat/skim
1 tsp vanilla extract
extra honey to drizzle

Directions:
Sauté honey in melted butter and stir in figs. Set aside.
Again, melt butter and sauté oats with a few figs and roast for five minutes.
Mix in milk and vanilla and boil.
Remove the pan from heat when the desired consistency is achieved.
Mix roasted figs and oats and serve.

Nutrition Info: Calories:296 kcal Fat:7 g Protein: 6.3g Carbs:29.3 g Fiber: 3.3g

Breakfast spanakopita

Preparation time:10 minutes
Cooking time: minutes
Servings: 2

Ingredients:

1 tbsp butter
4 oz Spinach
1 oz feta cheese
Two green onions
Four eggs
1/4 tsp black pepper
1/2 tsp dill weed
1 oz cheese
1 tbsp chives

Directions:

In a medium skillet, melt the butter. Add the dill, onions, and spinach, occasionally stirring.

In a container, combine the feta, eggs, dill, cream cheese, and pepper. Transfer the mixture in a skillet over the spinach. Toss and cook for a few minutes.

Serve and enjoy it.

Nutrition Info: Calories:288 kcal Fat: 22g Protein:18 g Carbs:5.3 g Fiber: 1.8g

Stuffed figs

Preparation time: 10 minutes
Cooking time: 8 minutes
Servings: 6

Ingredients:
12 large figs
1/4 cup toasted walnuts
3-1/2 oz Cambozola cheese
Honey

Directions: Fill the fig with Cambozola and put it in a baking tray.
Bake in a preheated oven at 350 degrees for eight minutes.
Drizzle some walnuts and honey and serve.

Nutrition Info: Calories: 203kcal Fat:8 g Protein: 5g Carbs:31 g Fiber: 4g

Vegetable breakfast bowl

Preparation time: 10 minutes
Cooking time: 50 minutes
Servings: 3

Ingredients:
One breakfast veggie sausage patty
One egg
1/2 oz cheddar cheese
½ cup roasted veggies
optional mix-ins: tomatoes, herbs, spinach, avocado

Directions: Bake veggies in a preheated oven at 425 degrees for 45 minutes.
Crack eggs and add cheese.
Mix them all and serve.

Nutrition Info: Calories:420 kcal Fat:31 g Protein: 24g Carbs:12 g Fiber:1 g

Breakfast green smoothie

Preparation time:5 minutes

Cooking time: 0minutes

Servings: 1

Ingredients:

2 tbsp hemp hearts

2 cup spinach

One medium banana

2 cup pineapple

1/2 an apple

2 cups of water

Directions: Blend all the items in the blender and serve.

Nutrition Info: Calories: 229kcal Fat: 4.6g Protein:4.7 g Carbs: 48g Fiber: g

Simple and quick steak

Preparation time: 20minutes
Cooking time: minutes
Servings: 2

Ingredients:
2 tbsp butter
1/2 tsp minced garlic
1 tsp minced parsley
1/4 tsp soy sauce
1/8 tsp salt
One beef steak
1/8 tsp pepper

Directions: Mix garlic, sauce, butter, and parsley. The garlic butter sauce is ready.
Cook steak in heated butter over medium flame for eight minutes.

Nutrition Info: Calories: 316kcal Fat:20 g Protein: 32g Carbs: 0g Fiber:0 g

Vegetable stew

Preparation time: 3 minutes
Cooking time: 15 minutes
Servings: 1

Ingredients:
1 tsp olive oil
One chopped sweet onion
1 tsp minced garlic
Two chopped zucchinis
One diced red bell pepper
Two chopped carrots
Black pepper to taste
Two cups of broccoli florets
2 cups low sodium vegetable stock
Two chopped large tomatoes
1 tsp of ground coriander
Half tsp of ground cumin
black pepper up to taste
2 tbsp of chopped fresh cilantro
Cayenne pepper

Directions:
Heat the olive oil on moderate heat in a saucepan
Add garlic & onion till softened about 3 min.

Add carrots, bell pepper, and zucchini. Sauté it until softened for almost 5 min.

Stir in vegetable stock, coriander, tomatoes, broccoli, and cayenne pepper. Cook until boiled and then reduce heat. Simmer until vegetables are tendered and stir for 5 min. Season the dish with pepper & serve hot with cilantro.

Nutrition Info: Calories: 286 kcal Fat: 7 g Protein: 7 g Carbs: 48 g Fiber: 7 g

Hot curry powder

Preparation time: 5 minutes
Cooking time: 0 minute
Servings: 2

Ingredients:

¼ cup ground coriander

3 tbsp turmeric

¼ cup ground cumin

½ tsp ground cloves

½ tbsp green chili powder

2 tsp ground cardamom

2 tbsp sweet paprika

2 tbsp ground mustard

1 tbsp fennel powder

1 tsp ground cinnamon

Directions:

Put the cumin, paprika, coriander, green chili powder, turmeric, mustard, cinnamon, fennel powder, cardamom, & cloves in the blender, & pulse until the ingredients are ground & well mixed. Put the curry powder into a small container with a lid. Store in a cool & dry place for six months.

Nutrition Info: Calories: 5 kcal Fat: 2 g Protein:g Carbs: 10 g Fiber: 0.1 g

Low sodium mayonnaise

Preparation time: 10 minutes
Cooking time: 0 minute
Servings: 1

Ingredients:
Two egg yolks
1 tsp honey
2 cups of olive oil
2 tbsp white vinegar
1 tsp Dijon mustard
2 tbsp of fresh lemon juice

Directions:
Whisk the yolks, mustard, vinegar, honey, & lemon juice. Whisk in the olive oil until all the oil is utilized & the mayonnaise becomes thick.
Use a sealed glass container to store in the refrigerator for two weeks.

Nutrition Info: Calories: 126 kcal Fat: 14 g Protein: 0 g Carbs: 0 g Fiber: 0 g

Green breakfast soup

Preparation time: 8 minutes
Cooking time: 4 minutes
Servings: 1

Ingredients:
2 cups spinach
2 cup vegetable stock
1 tsp ground coriander
½ avocado
Black pepper to taste
1 tsp cumin
1 tsp turmeric

Directions: Put all the ingredients in a blender and continue to grind until smooth
Transfer the ground mixture to a saucepan and cook until 2-3 minutes. Soup is ready

Nutrition Info: Calories: 95 kcal Fat: 3.8 g Protein: 3 g Carbs: 13.2 g Fiber: 3.1 g

Creamy broccoli soup

Preparation time: 5 minutes
Cooking time: 20 minutes
Servings: 3

Ingredients:

2 cups chopped broccoli
1 tsp olive oil
half roughly chopped sweet onion
4 cups vegetable broth
¼ cup grated parmesan cheese
black pepper
1 cup of rice milk

Directions:

Heat the olive oil in a medium saucepan over high heat. Add the onion & cook for 3-5 min, until onion begins to soften. Add broccoli & broth. Season it with pepper.
Bring a boil & reduce the heat. Then simmer uncovered for 10 min, until broccoli is tendered but bright green.
Now put the soup mixture into a blender. Add rice milk & process until smooth. Now put in the saucepan, add some parmesan cheese & serve.

Nutrition Info: Calories: 243 kcal Fat: 12.7 g Protein: 10.5 g Carbs: 25.4 g Fiber: 504 g

Roasted root vegetables

Preparation time: 5 minutes
Cooking time: 30 minutes
Servings: 3

Ingredients:

1 cup Chopped rutabaga

1 cup Chopped parsnips

1 cup Chopped turnips

1 tbsp olive oil

black pepper up to taste

1 tsp fresh chopped rosemary

Directions:

Preheat oven up to 400°F.

Toss the turnips and all the other ingredients in a large bowl. Bake the vegetables until they are tendered & browned (20-25 min) & stirring once.

Nutrition Info: Calories: 137 kcal Fat: 7.1 g Protein: 2.9 g Carbs: 17.2 g Fiber: 5 g

Spinach falafel wrap

Preparation time: 10 minutes
Cooking time: 8 minutes
Servings: 2

Ingredients:
15 oz of chickpeas
One small spinach
¾ cup Flour
2 tsp ground cumin.
¼ cup Plain yogurt
Two minced garlic cloves
black pepper according to taste
2 tbsp of canola oil for frying.
Four tortillas
One cucumber
green salad for serving
One lemon
Two slices of red onion

Directions:
Put spinach in a colander. Place it into the sink & pour the boiling water on it to wilt the spinach. Then allow it to cool and press as possible so that the water is squeezed from spinach. Add spinach, cumin, chickpeas, and flour to the food processor. Pulse until the mixture is just blended.

Make balls from the mixture.

Heat 1 tbsp of oil. Add ½ of falafel patties & cook for 2-3 min from each side, until they are browned & crisp. Repeat the process with remaining.

Combine yogurt, lemon juice, pepper & garlic in a bowl.

Place two patties in every tortilla and some cucumber spears, then some red onion and green salad ring. Use 1 tbsp of plain yogurt sauce for topping.

Nutrition Info: Calories: 274 kcal Fat: 10 g Protein: 8 g Carbs: 35 g Fiber: 8 g

Vegetable biryani

Preparation time: 10 minutes
Cooking time: 35 minutes
Servings: 2

Ingredients:
1 cup Basmati rice
2 tbsp of olive oil
1 tsp curry powder
1 tsp cumin seeds
1 tsp coriander seeds
2 cups of water
Chopped onion- half
Two minced garlic cloves
1 tbsp ground coriander
1/2 tsp cardamom
1 tsp cumin
1/4 tsp turmeric
2 cups cauliflower florets
1 cup cut green beans
one diced carrot.
¼ cup of chopped cilantro leaves

Directions:
Rinse the rice till the clear water runs & drain.

Heat 1 tbsp of olive oil on moderate heat & add curry powder coriander seeds & cumin seeds until they begin to give fragrance. Then add rice in the heating pot with 1¾ water cups. Heat until boil & then reduce the heat cover & simmer them for 12 min. Then off the stove. Cover for 10 min and steam.

And now heat olive oil (remaining tbsp) in another pot. Add onions & cook (6-8 min) until they give a golden look. Then add garlic & cook for one extra min. add cumin, coriander, turmeric, and cardamom and continue stirring until it is fragrant for about one minute.

Add carrots, cauliflower, and beans and cook (2-3 min). Then add the remaining 2/3rd cup of water into the pan, cover it & cook for 7-10 min till vegetables are just tendered.

Add the rice to vegetables & stir to blend. Top with cilantro leaves & serve.

Nutrition Info: Calories: 393 kcal Fat: 7 g Protein: 7 g Carbs: 72 g Fiber: 4 g

Greek couscous salad

Preparation time: 10 minutes
Cooking time: 0 minute
Servings: 2

Ingredients:

¼ cup of low sodium feta cheese
Three cups of cooked couscous.
One cup of cherry tomatoes
One chopped scallion, green & white parts.
One Eng. Diced cucumber.
Half a cup of black olives.
2 tbsp of fresh chopped parsley.
One tbsp of fresh lemon juice.
2 tbsp of balsamic vinegar

Directions:

Mix all the ingredients in a large bowl.
Top it with the feta cheese & the salad is ready to serve

Nutrition Info: Calories: 326 kcal Fat: 10 g Protein: 17 g Carbs: 51 g Fiber: 6 g

German braised cabbage

Preparation time: 15-20 min

Cooking time: 15 min

Servings: 1

Ingredients:
1 tbsp of olive oil

One-fourth chopped sweet onion.

Five cups of shredded red cabbage.

One pear, peeled & chopped

3 tbsp of vinegar.

Half tsp dry mustard.

One tbsp of sugar.

Half tsp caraway seeds.

Directions: Heat olive oil on moderate heat in a frying pan. Add cabbage, onion & pear. sauté till tendered for 10 min. Stir together vinegar, caraway seed sugar & mustard in a bowl. Combine cabbage and vinegar mixture and stir. Cover for 5 min. Now serve hot.

Nutrition Info: 94 Calories: kcal Fat: 3 g Protein: 2 g Carbs: 15 g Fiber: 3 g

Vibrant carrot soup

Preparation time:10 minutes
Cooking time: 20-25 minutes
Servings: 1-2

Ingredients:
1 tbsp of olive oil
Half chopped onion.
2 tsp of fresh ginger.
One tsp of fresh minced garlic
4 cups of water
Three chopped carrots.
1 tsp turmeric powder.
Half cup of coconut milk
One tbsp of fresh chopped cilantro

Directions: Heat the olive oil in a saucepan on medium heat. Sauté onion, garlic & ginger till softened 3 min.
Stir in water, carrots & turmeric. Bring a boil & reduce heat and simmer till the carrots are tendered (20 min).
Transfer soup in a blender along with coconut milk and pulse until soup becomes smooth.
Serve the soup topped with cilantro.

Nutrition Info: Calories: 113, kcal Fat: 10 g Protein: 2 g Carbs: 8 g Fiber: 2g

Open-faced bagel breakfast sandwich

Preparation time: 10 minutes
Cooking time: 10-15 minutes
Servings: 2

Ingredients:
one halved multigrain bagel.
Two tbsp divided cream cheese.
Two slices of tomato
One slice of red onion
black pepper
One cup of microgreens.

Directions: Light toast bagel in an oven or toaster.
Spread one tbsp of cheese on each bagel halves.
Top each half with one tomato slice & a couple of onion rings and season with black pepper.
Now top each half with a half cup of microgreens. Now it is ready to serve.

Nutrition Info: Calories: 164, kcal Fat: 6g, Protein: 6g: Carbs: 23g: Fiber: 3g

Rigatoni with emerald sauce

Preparation time: 10 minutes
Cooking time: 20-30 minutes
Servings: 2

Ingredients:
260 g kale
One clove of garlic.
4 oz of olive oil.
Twelve ounces of rigatoni.
One and a half tbsp of freshly grated parmesan.
¼ tsp of black pepper.

Directions:
Remove the stalk from kale leaves.
Blanch the leaves into the boiling water along with garlic clove for draining up to 3 min.
Take a food processor and put kale & garlic into it & blend to puree. Pour the olive oil in it & process until it becomes smooth.
Cook rigatoni according to the direction given in the package.
Place pasta into a bowl & add the sauce to it. Mix it well.
Divide this into the bowls for serving and add parmesan cheese over it. Top it with black pepper.

Nutrition Info: Calories: 414, kcal Fat: 30 g Protein: 7g Carbs: 30g Fiber: 2g

Korean mushroom bibimbap

Preparation time: 25 minutes

Cooking time: 25-30 minutes

Servings: 4

Ingredients:

BIBIMBAP

1 cup of Japanese rice

One and a half tbsp of olive oil

Four ounces of thin-sliced oyster mushrooms.

4 ounces of sliced cremini mushrooms

Half cucumber peeled and sliced.

Coating Spray thin.

Four eggs

one grated garlic clove.

1 cup spinach.

Two tsp of Japanese seaweed.

Sriracha sauce (optional)

Gochujang paste (optional)

1/4 cup of sprouts, any type (optional)

DRESSING

1 ½ tbsp of Japanese low sodium soy sauce.

1 tbsp of sesame oil

1 tbsp of rice vinegar

2 tsp of honey

Directions:

Cook the rice according to the direction given by the package

Heat 1 tbsp of olive oil on moderate heat.

Sauté mushrooms for 5 min.

Lower the heat. Add additional half tbsp olive oil seven cooks for more than 10 minutes.

Combine all ingredients for the dressing.

Pour 1/2 of dressing over cucumbers in a small bowl.

Heat one separate small pan over moderate heat with cooking spray. Now cook the egg according to your wish.

Add the garlic & the spinach into mushrooms. Sauté for 2 min till the spinach wilts. Continue stirring

pour remaining dressing on the cooked vegetables & mix well.

Divide the rice into four individual serving bowls. Arrange the mushroom mixture, cucumber & sprouts on the rice.

Top every bowl with one cooked egg.

Garnish using Japanese seasoning.

Add a dollop of sriracha sauce for additional flavor. Top with the sprouts.

Nutrition Info: Calories:350 kcal Fat:13 g Protein: 10 g Carbs: 47g Fiber: 3g

Bulgur wheat salad with pomegranate molasses chicken

Preparation time: 15 minutes
Cooking time: 10 minutes
Servings: 4

Ingredients:

One small red onion, thinly sliced

100 g feta, crumbled

2 tbsp mint, thinly shredded

2 x 250 g bulgur wheat, chickpeas, and quinoa

2½ tbsp pomegranate molasses

40 g chopped pistachios

460 g chicken breasts

1 tsp sunflower oil

50 g pomegranate seeds

Directions:

Preheat oven to 400 F. Take an ovenproof frying pan and heat the oil in it over medium heat. Season the chicken breasts with spices and fry them for 2-3 minutes on both sides in the pan. Retract the pan off the fire and sprinkle 1½ tablespoons of pomegranate molasses with the chicken. Transfer to oven and cook until the mixture is fully cooked, for about 8 minutes or. Take out of the oven and allow for a couple of minutes to rest.

Meanwhile, following the directions on the box, cook the grains. Mix with the feta, mint, red onion, and pomegranate seeds. Divide the mixture of grains into four serving plates. Cut the chicken and the leftover pomegranate molasses, pass to the dishes, and drizzle. To toast, cover with pistachios.

Nutrition Info: Calories: 198 kcal Fat: 17 g Protein: 44.5 g Carbs: 7.8 g Fiber: 7.8 g

Broccoli and Capsicum Pasta Salad

Preparation time: 8 hours 30 minutes
Cooking time: 20 minutes
Servings: 6

Ingredients:

350 g broccoli florets
280 g radiator pasta
175 g yellow or red grape tomatoes
One yellow zucchini, thinly sliced
One red onion, chopped
One large sliced red capsicum
Dressing
20 g chopped fresh parsley
80 ml of olive oil
150 ml cider vinegar
2 tbsp chopped fresh dill
pepper to taste

Directions:

1. Put out a big iced water cup. Over a high flame, put a big saucepan of water to a boil. In a broad metal sieve, placed the broccoli, red capsicum, onion, and zucchini. Immerse and blanch in the pool for about 2 minutes or before the shades brighten. Drain and lift, then dive into the cold sea.

2. In a saucepan of boiling water, cook the pasta according to the package directions. Drain and position in a large bowl for serving. Wash the vegetables and add them and also the tomatoes to the pasta.

3. lace the vinegar, oil, dill, parsley, and pepper in a container with a tight-fitting lid to make the seasoning, and shake until fully mixed. To coat, pour on the salad and toss gently. For at least 8 hours or overnight, cover and refrigerate. Until serving, toss again.

Nutrition Info: Calories: 270 kcal Fat: 11 g Protein: 22 g Carbs: 34 g Fiber: 2 g

Sesame Salad Dressing

Preparation time: 3 minutes
Cooking time: 3 minutes
Servings: 1

Ingredients:
1/4 cup olive oil
1/4 cup soy sauce
1/4 cup white vinegar
1 1/2 tbsp honey
2 tbsp toasted sesame oil

Directions:
1. In a container, put the ingredients and shake until the sugar dissolves. Change saltiness with the salt and sugar with sweetness to taste.
2. Leave it in the fridge for up to 3 weeks (to be safe). Take to room temperature and shake well before use.
3. For 3 to 4 cups of chopped cabbage or leafy greens, the side salad for four persons, a single serving dish is enough.

Nutrition Info: Calories: 52 kcal Fat: 5.8 g Protein: 0.2 g Carbs: 1.4 g Fiber: 1 g

Mediterranean Grain Salad

Preparation time: 5 minutes
Cooking time: 35 minutes
Servings: 1

Ingredients:
Coarse salt to taste
Black pepper 2 tsp olive oil 1/2 minced small shallot 1/2 cup parsley, chopped 1 tbsp red wine vinegar 1 oz goat cheese, crumbled 1 cup grape tomatoes, halved

Directions: Combine the bulgur with 1/4 tsp salt and 1 cup of boiling water in a heat-proof dish. Cover, and let rest for about 30 minutes, before tender but somewhat chewy.
Drain the bulgur and press to extract liquid in the fine-mesh sieve; return to the bowl. Add the onions, parsley, vinegar, shallot, and oil. Then season with pepper and salt, and toss. Top with cheese.

Nutrition Info: Calories:303 kcal Fat: 21g Protein: 10g Carbs: 21g Fiber: 4g

Macadamia Nut Dressing

Preparation time: 10 minutes

Cooking time: 10 minutes

Servings: 4

Ingredients:

¼ tsp onion powder

½ tsp pepper

1 cup Cashew Milk

1 cup Macadamia Nuts

1 tbsp chives, chopped

1 tbsp lemon juice

1 tsp apple cider vinegar

1 tsp garlic powder

1 tsp salt

2 tbsp parsley

Directions:

A high-powered mixer and places all the ingredients (other than green onions and chives, and parsley). Start at low and bring it up to high speed steadily until the ingredients are fully blended. If you want a thinner consistency, add more Homemade Cashew Milk from Nature's Eats. Add now the diced chives and parsley, then blend until smooth.Now serve promptly or store it in the refrigerator in an air-tight bag.

Nutrition Info: Calories: 302 kcal Fat: 26 g Protein: 8 g Carbs: 19 g Fiber: 6.3 g

Vinaigrette Dressing

Preparation time: 5 minutes
Cooking time: 5 minutes
Servings: 1

Ingredients:
black pepper, to taste
3 tbsp vinegar
Two cloves garlic, minced
1 tbsp honey
1 tbsp Dijon mustard
½ cup olive oil
¼ tsp salt

Directions:
Combine all the ingredients in a liquid mixing cup. With a small spoon or a fork, stir well till ingredients are thoroughly mixed together.
Now taste, and customize as needed. Thin it out with a little more olive oil if the mixture becomes too acidic, or balance the flavors with a bit more maple, honey, or syrup. Add a pinch of salt if the mixture is a bit blah. If the zing is not enough, apply a teaspoon of vinegar.
Serve instantly, or for potential use, cover, and refrigerate. For 7 to 10 days, the homemade vinaigrette lasts well. If the vinaigrette solidifies in the fridge somewhat, don't think about it. It helps to do this with real olive oil. Simply let it for 5 to 10 minutes at room temperature or microwave very quickly (approximately 20 secs) to liquefy that olive oil again. Now serve.

Nutrition Info: Calories: 183 kcal Fat: 19.1 g Protein: 0.4 g Carbs: 4.3 g Fiber: 0.2 g

Steamed Broccoli Salad

Preparation time: 10 minutes
Cooking time: 1 minute
Servings: 4-5

Ingredients:
1 tbsp red wine vinegar
1/3 cup olive oil
1/4 tsp black pepper
1/4 tsp red pepper flakes
2 tsp cumin seeds
2 tsp sesame oil, roasted
3/4 tsp salt
Four minced garlic cloves
1lb broccoli florets

Directions:
Cook raw broccoli: In the red wine vinegar, toss broccoli with salt and pepper. "Set aside for 10 minutes, the broccoli will be pickled gently, almost "ceviche.
Garlic, seasoning, and oil mix: Melt the oil over medium heat in a small skillet. Cumin seeds, garlic, and flakes of red pepper are added. Cook until the garlic is bright golden, stirring.
Broccoli toss: Dump the oil mix over the broccoli immediately. Using the rubber spatula to clean up the oil from all the bowl sides, throw very well.
Marinate: Leave to marinate for at least 1 hour, or refrigerate for 48 hours (it gets better over time).
For the best taste, serve at room temperature, not cold!

Nutrition Info: Calories: 18 kcal Fat: 17 g Protein: 3 g Carbs: 8 g Fiber: 3 g

Pomegranate Feta Salad

Preparation time: 10 minutes
Cooking time: 10 minutes
Servings: 3

Ingredients:
10 oz mixed baby greens
One pomegranate
8 oz crumbled feta cheese
1/2 cup pecans
1/4 cup granulated sugar
1/4 red onion, sliced
Dressing
salt to taste
pepper to taste
3 tbsp red wine vinegar
3 tbsp olive oil
1 tsp Dijon mustard
One lemon, zested and juiced

Directions:
Pour the sugar into a small skillet to form the candied pecans and pour pecans on top. Then cook until the sugar melts and gives a caramel color, stirring continuously over medium heat to not burn nuts and sugar. Have patience! The sugar takes a while to begin to melt.
When the sugar turns, keep stirring to cover the pecans with a caramel color coat. To cool, spill pecans on the greased wax paper/aluminum foil. Split them into pieces until the pecans are cooled.
Place (in a large mixing bowl) the lettuce, red onion, pomegranate seeds, pecan pieces, feta cheese, and set aside.

In a separate cup, mix the lemon zest, Dijon mustard, olive oil, vinegar, lemon juice, salt, and pepper. Pour the salad over and toss to cover it. Immediately serve now.

Nutrition Info: Calories: 147 kcal Fat: 7 g Protein: 3 g Carbs: 22 g Fiber: 3 g

Grated beetroot & carrot salad

Preparation time: 15 minutes
Cooking time: 0 minute
Servings: 4

Ingredients:
One pinch of salt
Pinch of cayenne
2 tsp honey
2 tbsp sliced mint leaves
2 tbsp lemon juice
2 cups of grated carrots (from about three carrots)
1/4 tsp ground cumin
1/4 tsp cinnamon
1/2 teaspoon paprika
1/2 cup golden raisins
1 cup of grated beets

Directions:
Drain the beetroot, mix with the carrots and raisins, and put the sliced carrots in the medium serving dish.
Put the grated beets in a sieve and rinse with cold water briefly. Drain away some of that extra beet juice that will make the entire salad beet red otherwise. Pat with a paper towel to rinse and add the carrots to the bowl for them. Add some raisins. Stir to mix softly.
Render the dressing: Mix the paprika, cinnamon, cumin, salt, and cayenne in a small cup. Then add the honey and lemon juice and mix until smooth.
Garnish with carrots and beets and let stay for an hour: scatter over the carrots & beets and fold softly until the carrots & beets are finely covered, either cooled or at the room temperature, for

an hour before eating, so that the dressing can seep into the beets and carrots.

Before eating, stir in sliced mint: Stir in a few teaspoons of sliced new mint leaves just before serving. Garnish the new mint with it.

Nutrition Info: Calories: 344 kcal Fat: 20 g Protein: 10.3 g Carbs: 34.7 g Fiber: 8 g

Roasted vegetable lentil salad

Preparation time: 10 minutes
Cooking time: 35 minutes
Servings: 4

Ingredients:
salt and pepper
Four carrots, chopped
4 tbsp hemp seeds
Two zucchinis, chopped
2 tbsp honey
2 tbsp balsamic vinegar
2 1/4 cups vegetable broth
One white onion, sliced
One sweet potato, cubed
1 tbsp rosemary
1 tbsp thyme
1 cup brown lentils

Directions:
Preheat the oven to 425°F.
Chop all the vegetables and scatter them in a single layer over the baking trays. Depending upon the scale, you can require 2 or 3 trays. Drizzle them in a large bowl with 1 tsp of olive oil (add all the sliced vegetables to a large bowl if it's simpler, toss with oil and spices, and then add to the bowls) and sprinkle with rosemary and thyme. Also, apply a touch of salt and pepper. Using the palms until they're well-coated and blend them all. For 35-40 minutes, roast the vegetables in the oven until soft and browned.
On the stovetop, boil the broth or water, add the lentils, and then cover and minimize the heat to a medium simmer. Cook until the lentils are soft, for 20-25 minutes.

Add everything to a big bowl and then toss with the maple syrup, balsamic vinegar, and hemp seeds until the lentils and veggies are cooked, or split the lentils, hemp seeds, and roasted vegetables between the four bowls or containers, then blend the maple syrup and balsamic vinegar in a small dish together and drizzle on each serving. If necessary, season with pepper and salt and serve right away.

Nutrition Info: Calories: 417 kcal Fat: 6 g Protein: 19 g Carbs: 76 g Fiber: 13 g

Herbed Quinoa and Pomegranate Salad

Preparation time: 20 minutes
Cooking time: 40 minutes
Servings: 8

Ingredients:
Salad
1/3 cup chopped fresh mint leaves
1/3 cup chopped fresh parsley leaves
1/3 cup dried cranberries or raisins
1/3 cup fresh pomegranate arils
1/3 cup slivered almonds
1/3 cup sliced Kalamata olives
1 cup quinoa
Dressing
Several twists of black pepper
¼ teaspoon salt
¼ teaspoon ground cinnamon
¼ cup olive oil
¼ cup lemon juice

Directions: To cook quinoa: First of all, rinse the quinoa for a minute or two under running water in a fine mesh colander. Merge the washed quinoa and 2 cups of water in a medium-sized bath. Bring the mixture to a boil, then cover the pan. Cook for about 15 minutes. Remove the quinoa from the heat and let it stay for 5 minutes, already wrapped. Uncover the pot, skim off any extra water, and use a fork to fluff the quinoa. Set it to cool aside.
To toast almonds: Heat the almonds on medium-low heat in a small skillet, constantly stirring, until fragrant and becoming golden on the edges. Let them not be charred! To cool, move the toasted almonds to a serving dish.

Mix the olive oil, salt, cinnamon, lemon juice, and frequent ground black pepper to make the dressing.

Final assembly: mix the quinoa, minced mint, and parsley, cranberries, pomegranate, and olives or cheese in your serving bowl in addition to almonds. Drizzle the salad with the dressing and toss to cover. If required, taste and blend in extra salt, pepper, and olive oil. Serve instantly or refrigerate until later.

Nutrition Info: Calories: 427 kcal Fat: 25.4 g Protein: 8.7 g Carbs: 45 g Fiber: 6.5 g

Salad Niçoise

Preparation time: 10 minutes
Cooking time: 20 minutes
Servings: 4

Ingredients:
salt and pepper to taste
8 cups mixed greens
Seven red potatoes, unpeeled
Three tomatoes, cubed
Two red peppers, roasted and sliced
Two boiled eggs, sliced
2 tbsp capers
2 tbsp canola oil
1/2 lb haricots vent
1/2 cup black olives
1 lb tuna
Vinaigrette dressing
salt and pepper to taste
3 tbsp white wine vinegar
2 tsp Dijon mustard
1/3 cup olive oil
1/2 shallot, minced
1/2 tsp sugar
1 tbsp lemon juice

Directions:
Spray both sides with pepper and salt to cook the tuna. Heat oil, preferably cast iron, in a large skillet over high heat. Add the tuna when the oil becomes very hot and mildly smoky. Sear for 2 minutes. On the one hand, flip the tuna and sear for around 1 min. Remove from the skillet and leave to rest on a cutting board.

In a big pot, add the potatoes and cover them with water. Add on a pair of teaspoons of salt. Carry to a boil, and simmer until the potatoes become cooked through, for about 15 minutes. Bring another container of water to a boil, add the green beans, turn off the heat, and rest for 2 minutes. Drain and coat the vegetables with cold water. Dry Pat.

To a platter or big shallow dish, add the greens. Thinly slice the salmon. Set the fish, potatoes, green beans, olives, capers, and tomatoes in rows.

Whisk together the lemon juice, vinegar, shallots, mustard, and garlic to make the vinaigrette. With salt and pepper, season. Whisk in the olive oil gently, in a thin stream, until emulsified. Drizzle over the salad with the dressing and eat.

Nutrition Info: Calories: 423 kcal Fat: 21 g Protein: 28 g Carbs: 22 g Fiber: 10 g

Roasted sweet potato and black bean salad

Preparation time: 10 minutes
Cooking time: 40 minutes
Servings: 4

Ingredients:
1 cup cooked black beans
One clove garlic, minced
1 lb sweet potatoes
One small red Onion
1/2 cup cilantro
1/2 tsp chili powder
1/4 cup pepitas
1/4 tsp salt
3 tbsp olive oil, divided
Juice and zest from 1 lime

Directions:
Preheat the oven to 400 degrees F. Peel the sweet potatoes, cut them into 1/4-inch pieces, and put them on a tray of sheets. Chop the onion and add it to the tray into 1/4-inch bits. Drizzle on top of 1 tablespoon olive oil and add 1/4 teaspoon salt.
Mix until the sweet potatoes are fully coated. Spread out into a single layer and cook for 35 to 40 minutes before the sweet potatoes are soft and start browning.
Combine the remaining two teaspoons of olive oil in a container with lime juice, one teaspoon of lime zest, chili powder, and minced garlic when roasting the sweet potatoes. Just shake good.
When the sweet potatoes are full, move them to a dish. Using the black beans, cilantro, and pepitas to throw in. Drizzle and

toss with the dressing before the salad is mixed. With the sweet potatoes still soft, this is best done.

Nutrition Info: Calories: 303 kcal Fat: 14.5 g Protein: 8.5 g Carbs: 15 g Fiber: 8.6 g

Cannellini Bean Soup

Preparation time: 5 minutes
Cooking time: 20 minutes
Servings: 4

Ingredients:
Two sliced potatoes
2 cups vegetable broth
Two cans of cannellini beans
1-2 diced garlic cloves
1/8 tsp black pepper
1/3 cup white wine
1/2 tsp paprika
1/2 tsp salt
1 tbsp tomato paste
1 tbsp olive oil
One sprig rosemary
One diced onion
One diced carrot
1 cup spinach
One diced celery stalk

Directions:
Heat the olive oil over medium heat in a big kettle. Add the diced celery, carrot, and onion until the oil shimmers. Cook for about 5 minutes, stirring regularly until the onion is soft and turns translucent.
Add the potatoes, tomato paste, beans, garlic, rosemary (whatever is better for you, the whole sprig, sliced, or dried), and paprika. (If you use it). (if you use it). (if you use it). (if you use it). (if you use it). (if you use it). Cook for about 1 minute, stirring constantly.

Pour in the wine, mix well, and let it boil for another minute until it has evaporated.

Then include frozen spinach in the vegetables' broth and a pleasant pinch of salt & pepper. Boost the heat, boil the mixture, gently cover the kettle, and reduce the heat and simmer for 15 minutes.

Remove the pot from the heat until the potatoes are soft and the soup is dense and fluffy, then remove the rosemary sprig*. Taste and season with pepper and salt. Based on the vegetable broth or your preferences, you can need more salt.

Break into cups, drizzle with extra virgin olive oil or olive oil, and add more ground black pepper as you prefer. Serve with the crusty whole-grain bread, and add fresh parmesan cheese for extra spice if you do not keep it vegan. Enjoy! Enjoy!

Nutrition Info: Calories: 350 kcal Fat: 1 g Protein: 19 g Carbs: 57 g Fiber: 13 g

Garlic, sweet potato, and chickpea soup

Preparation time: 10 minutes
Cooking time: 30 minutes
Servings: 4-6

Ingredients:
lemon juice
Eight cloves garlic, sliced
400 g chickpeas
350 g cooked sweet potato
30 g olive oil
2 tsp ground turmeric
2 tsp dried thyme
1 tsp salt
One chopped onion
½ tsp cayenne pepper

Directions: In a big saucepan with water, place the garlic, olive oil, and onions: this produces more steam to rapidly tender the garlic. Then bring the fire to a boil and simmer for five min until the water evaporates and the garlic is very tender.
Add the sweet potatoes, salt, thyme, turmeric, chickpeas, cayenne, and 800 ml of water, and bring to a boil until the sweet potatoes have further softened. Remove from the sun and slightly cool off.
In a mixer, puree the mixture until creamy. If necessary, return to the pan, change the consistency with additional water, and then heat it until it boils. Divide between 4 and 6 bowls and apply a drizzle of lemon juice and a few shreds of black pepper to each bowl.

Nutrition Info: Calories: 407 kcal Fat: 11 g Protein: 13.4 g Carbs: 41 g Fiber: 9.7 g

Kumara, coconut, and lemongrass soup

Preparation time: 10 minutes
Cooking time: 25 minutes
Servings: 6

Ingredients:
One chopper White onion
5 cups of Vegetable Stock
Thai Basil - for garnish
2 lb chopped Sweet Potatoes
2 tbsp Olive Oil
2 Lemongrass Stalks
2 Kaffir Lime Leaves
½ tsp chopped ginger
½ tbsp Chopped garlic
½ cup Coconut Milk
Four chopped Celery Stalks

Directions:
On a moderate flame, heat the olive oil. Sweat until the onion is transparent, the chopped onion, ginger, lemongrass, garlic, lime leaves, and celery.
Add in the vegetable supply and sweet potatoes. Carry to a boil, reduce the heat until it is cooked and then simmer cover for around 25 min or until the sweet potatoes are softened.
Now give a minute for the soup to cool off. Please cut the lime leaves and the lemongrass before you mix it into a smooth broth. Move all the ingredients carefully into your blender or cream the soup with a handheld blender.
Put the soup back in a clean dish, reheat, and add the milk from the coconut. Taste the broth and season with white pepper and some salt, if possible.

Reheat the soup before eating, put it in bowls, and spread some Thai basil on top.

Nutrition Info: Calories: 324 kcal Fat: 11 g Protein: 3 g Carbs: 49 g Fiber: 8 g

Moroccan Chickpea Soup

Preparation time: 15 minutes
Cooking time: 30 minutes
Servings: 3

Ingredients:
coriander sprigs
500 ml of vegetable stock
40 g seed mix, roasted
410 g tin chickpeas
400 g chopped tomatoes
1 tsp cumin seeds
1 tbsp olive oil
One chopped red pepper
One chopped onion
One crushed garlic clove
One chopped carrot

Directions: Heat the oil over medium heat in a saucepan, then add the seeds of onion, carrot, garlic, pepper, and cumin and fry for around 5 minutes. Stir in the stock and the tomatoes, and cook for 5 minutes.
Using a hand blender to purée the onions, stir in chickpeas, and heat them for 2 minutes.
Adorn with coriander/beans. With bread, serve.

Nutrition Info: Calories: 524 kcal Fat: 13.3 g Protein: 15.8 g Carbs: 38.5 g Fiber: 14 g

Ribollita

Preparation time: 15 minutes
Cooking time: 25 minutes
Servings: 10

Ingredients:
1 1/2 tsp salt
14 oz crushed tomatoes
One red onion, chopped
1 lb chopped cavolo nero
1/2 lb loaf of bread
Two chopped carrots
Three cloves garlic, chopped
3 tbsp olive oil
Four celery stalks, chopped
4 cups white beans, cooked
chopped black olives
1/2 tsp red pepper flakes
zest of one lemon

Directions:
Mix the olive oil, garlic, carrot, celery, and red onion in the largest dense pot over medium heat. Sweat the vegetables for 10 -15 minutes, but stop further browning. Add the tomatoes and flakes of red pepper and cook for another ten minutes, long enough to make the tomatoes thicken a little. Add the cavolo

nero, and 8 cups of water, 3 cups of beans, per 2 liters. Bring it to a boil, reduce the heat and cook for around 15 minutes until the greens are tender.

Meanwhile, with a generous splash of water, mash or puree the remaining beans - till smooth. Tear the bread into chunks. Add the bread and the beans to the soup. Simmer, stirring regularly, for 20 minutes or so, before the bread disintegrates and the soup becomes thick. Add the salt, taste and if appropriate, add more. Stir in the zest of the lemon.

Serve instantly, or cool overnight and refrigerate. With a bit of olive oil and some chopped olives, finish each serving.

Nutrition Info: Calories: 229 kcal Fat: 5 g Protein: 5 g Carbs: 4 g Fiber: 6 g

Broccoli soup

Preparation time: 10 minutes
Cooking time: 25 minutes
Servings: 6

Ingredients:

One onion, chopped
One stalk celery, chopped
2 cups of milk
3 cups chicken broth
3 tbsp all-purpose flour
5 tbsp butter, divided
8 cups broccoli florets
black pepper to taste

Directions:

In a medium-sized stock container, heat two tablespoons of butter and sauté the celery and onion until tender. Add the broccoli and broth, then cover for 10 minutes and simmer. In a mixer, pour the broth, filling the pitcher but no more than halfway full. With the folded kitchen towel, keep the blender's lid down and start the blender carefully, using a few short pulses to transfer the soup before leaving it to puree. Purée until smooth and dump into a clean pot in batches. Alternately, right in the frying pot, you should use a stick blender to puree the broth. Melt three tablespoons of butter over medium heat in a shallow saucepan, whisk in the flour and add the cream. Stir until bubbly and thick, and apply to the broth. Season and eat with pepper.

Nutrition Info: Calories: 207 kcal Fat: 12 g Protein: 9.2 g Carbs: 17 g Fiber: 3.6 g

Mushroom soup

Preparation time: 5 minutes
Cooking time: 45 minutes
Servings: 6

Ingredients:

Salt to taste

Black pepper to taste

Six sprigs thyme

4 cups chicken stock

3 tbsp olive oil

1/4 cup whipping cream

1/4 cup Cognac

1/4 cup chopped chives

1/2 cup minced shallot

One sprig rosemary

1 lb mixed mushrooms

1 lb cremini mushrooms

Directions:

Chop the mushroom stems roughly and let them simmer and covered for about an hour in the chicken broth. In a large skillet, heat the oil and sauté each shallot until they are transparent. Lightly add the spices, salt, and pepper. Chop the mushroom caps beautifully and precisely into the 1/2-inch dice. Add them as they are sliced into the shallots. Keep the heat very low until the mushroom fluid is released and then reabsorbed, and cook gently. Shake the cup so that they do not stick. Remove the rosemary and thyme. Turn the heat up, then add the Cognac. Flame it up if you just feel like Chef-y. Cook down the mushroom cap or shallot mixture until well-reduced and begin to turn the edges a bit golden.

Strain the fungus from the broth of the chicken. To the filtered broth, apply the wonderful shallot mixture and mushroom cap and heat it gently. Swirl in and serve the cream and chives. Or serve, if you like to get fancy, in tiny sipping bowls topped with chives and softly whipped cream.

Nutrition Info: Calories: 97 kcal Fat: 4 g Protein: 9 g Carbs: 6 g Fiber: 3 g

Guacamole

Preparation time: 10 minutes
Cooking time: 10 minutes
Servings: 4

Ingredients:

½ cup diced Onion

One lime, juiced

One pinch of cayenne pepper

1 tsp minced garlic

1 tsp salt

2 Roma tomatoes, diced

Three mashed avocados

3 tbsp chopped cilantro

Directions:

Mash the avocados along with lime juice and salt in a medium cup.

Combine the cilantro, tomato, onion, and garlic. Stir in the pepper with cayenne. For the best taste, refrigerate for 1 hour or serve it immediately.

Nutrition Info: Calories: 261.5 kcal Fat: 22.2 g Protein: 3.7 g Carbs:18 g Fiber: 11.4 g

Mushroom & Cardamom, Squash Soup

Preparation time: 8 minutes
Cooking time: 30 minutes
Servings: 3

Ingredients:

1 tsp ginger

One leek

1 tsp Celtic sea salt

125 ml of coconut cream

200 g mushrooms

250 ml passata

300 ml of water

350g of peeled squash

Four cardamom pods

1 cup herbs

Dash of coconut oil

Directions:

In a bowl, sugar, milk, salt, ginger, and past, cardamom into a squash. Cook and for 15 minutes. Blend the mixture. Sauté mushrooms in heated oil for five minutes. Serve in serving dish by making layers and serve.

Nutrition Info: Calories: 189 kcal Fat: 18.8 g Protein: 3.6 g Carbs: 4.7 g Fiber: 1.6 g

www.ingramcontent.com/pod-product-compliance
Lightning Source LLC
Chambersburg PA
CBHW070733030426
42336CB00013B/1962